Why you
need sleep!

Why you need sleep (Introduction)

Sleep is a strange beast. Despite DECADES of study, there's still so much we don't know about it.

The sleep cycle was only really discovered in the 1930's, and the four stages of that cycle were identified years later. And even though research continues, the sleep cycle proves largely impervious to the tamperings of modern medicine.

Sure, there are pills to make you sleep sooner, longer, or with fewer dreams, but none of them really make your sleep BETTER, or at least not without side effects.

Luckily, you don't actually need fancy pharmaceuticals to sleep well every night! Instead, you can rely on simple habits and a few powerful lifestyle changes. When all else fails, there are a few natural remedies that will improve your sleep health and help get you on the right night-time track.

Look, I get it:

There could be any number of reasons you might not be getting a great night's sleep. It might be as simple as drinking caffeine too late in the day- your last cup should be at least eight hours before bed- or as complex as a mood disorder. Identifying the reasons you aren't sleeping well is a vital step in improving your rest.

And that's what this book is all about. This is based on a lot of researching how to sleep better, sleep hacks, and methods that you can use TONIGHT to sleep better, and feel better in the morning.

You don't have to read this all the way through the first time, and many people will probably read a section here and there. *It's arranged into 50 tips, techniques and hacks for sleeping better, along with some bonus material at the end.*

But why is sleep important?

Sleep affects almost every process and system in your body and mind. It's absolutely essential for our survival and it helps us do all sorts of amazing things.

Specifically though, it multiplies any force you're trying to put out. If you're trying to achieve something whether it's becoming an athlete, writing a book or creating some art, getting better sleep will make it easier.

Sleep helps us recover from injury or exercise, it rejuvenates our minds and helps us think faster. It's pretty important, but most of us don't give it the attention or respect it deserves.

We're busy, we think we have to work during the night, and we keep ourselves awake at night with films and phone screens.

In the perfect world, we should be waking up when the sun rises in the morning, and going to sleep soon after it sets at night..

But how many people do that?

You'd be laughed at if you went to bed at 8:30PM in most social circles, but as we'll explore, it's important for a huge number of reasons.

This isn't as much a guide as it is a collection of useful tips and tricks you can use to sleep better. We've written this with the busy person in mind, so you can pick it up whenever you have a spare 5 minutes and just bite off a small section. Maybe you can just read one tip a day, and put it into practice! Let's go!

Technology and sleep

1: Technology and sleep (love/hate!)

One of the most common reasons people lose sleep in today's society is their technology.

Phones for example, make our lives simpler in many ways. We can talk to anyone at any time. Texting and instant messaging make communication simple and immediate.

Calendars, emails, jobs, games...everything is available. However, that constant access also creates a new expectation of constant availability:

You never get to "turn off."

Many people also use their phones as their alarms, so whenever they wake up, they check their phone for the time and get pulled in by the many notifications on their phone instantly.

Change up your technology habits for a better night's sleep. It might not be easy and there will certainly be pressure from all your iPhone apps and desktop bookmarks to consume more content, for longer, more often but TRY and break the cycle!

The best way of starting to do this is to separate your phone from your alarm clock. Buy a cheap alarm clock online and leave your phone in another room. This will help you think about it less, and not worry so much about notifications in the middle of the night. Even if your phone is on silent, you'll still THINK about checking it if you KNOW it's under your pillow.

And this leads to bad sleep habits, so put it in another room, and use an actual alarm clock to wake up. It makes a big difference! And you'll be able to wake up slowly and peacefully, maybe even say good morning to your partner first as well!

Lots of people often say they 'have' to use their phone as their alarm, but I would disagree. There's no special alarm function on a phone that you can't get on a real alarm clock, it's just an excuse. Try it for a few nights! Put your phone on to charge either across the room or in a totally different room of the house.

You could even go one step further with this, and just avoid social media entirely as well. Social media is a tool used to keep up with your friends and see what people are up to. It sounds good in theory, but what's actually going on?

Well, you likely don't even USE it for that any more.

The amount of adverts on big social media platforms has risen steadily month on month for years. If you really take a moment to scroll through and LOOK at what content you're being shown, most of it is adverts, and videos from pages you didn't even follow.

You rarely use it to actually share your life, and even when people do, it's a fake version. It's the 'best' version, the version of your life that looks best for the camera, for the 'likes'. It's rarely about your actual life, and everyone's just scrolling through these social media websites not really concerned with WHAT they're being shown.

It's because social media is addictive. The chemicals we get in our bodies when we scroll through or get attention on one of our posts are addictive. So that's why we keep coming back, but I challenge you to go a week without looking at social media.

I gave up all social media years ago, and it was the best thing I've done! I don't concern myself with adverts, or low vibration things like gossip and drama. I just focus on my life, the people I love, and experiencing the moment.

Removing blue light from screens

2: Removing blue light from screens

One easy change you can make, is to use a blue light cancelling app when you use your phone or tablet before bedtime.

There are also apps that allow you to read with a 'bluelight filter'.

Many of these will make your phone screen seem orange or yellow, but this is a good thing (although it takes some getting used to). Some tablets, like Kindles even come with built-in blue light filters, and you can set a schedule so that it always turns on when you're nearing bedtime.

Bluelight is a recent topic of many academic studies. They're finding that blue light actually changes the frequency of your brain waves. When you're getting close to sleep, your brain waves get longer and slightly slower.

Blue light entering the eyes actually causes your brainwaves to shorten, as though you are still AWAKE.

Blue light refers to the bright blue light emitted from things like TV screens, LED lights, phone screens etc. It's not actually needed for you to be able to see a picture on the screen though, which means you can turn it off, or down!

By cancelling out this blue light, you can avoid this shift in your brain wave length and stay on track for deep, quality sleep. You need those long brain waves to reach all of the four stages of the sleep cycle.

Think of the blue light in your screens like an artificial 'sun'.

Although it's nowhere near as powerful, because it's so harsh and artificial it DOES release the same hormones in your body that sun releases.

This means it keeps your body tuned to being awake. It stops you being able to relax, wind down, and start producing more 'sleep hormones' like melatonin.

Luckily, it's very easy to change this, and you can download or use apps and functions to stop blue light after certain times of the day. I use Fl.ux (not a typo, that's the name of the program) which works with Windows or Mac. It works on a timer, and once you've told it your wake up and bedtimes, it automatically takes the blue light down in the evenings.

You won't really notice it until it gets to about 9PM and the screen looks noticeably redder, but it has an enormous impact on your sleep! You'll be able to look at your laptop screen almost right up until bed time without it affecting your sleep too much.

Now, that being said I still wouldn't suggest looking at a screen right up to bed time. I'd suggest turning screens off at last an hour before bed, but we'll come to that later. If your work involves looking at screens at night or something like that, this is useful!

Another big hack you can use is to actually use the night mode on your phone. If you have an Iphone or modern Android phone, you can go into the settings and put night mode on after a certain time. This should remove the blue light as well.

There are blue light blocking glasses you can buy, but these are largely useless these days. Most technology comes built in with the ability to turn down blue light, so the glasses aren't really needed, but they're an option!

One thing to notice about this, is that you'll become very accustomed to the red light after a while. I've had friends come over and look at my laptop screen in the evenings, and they can't actually see the screen properly! People are so used to the blue light that we can't focus on a screen without it.

But after a few months, I adjusted to this change in colour and I'm able to easily see the screen and the details on it, even with very low brightness and no blue light. This change happens slowly over time.

So for the first few weeks of doing this, expect to find it a little bit harder to see the details on your screens. This is just because your eyes have never had to adjust to see things this way. It gets much easier with every day that you do it.

Video games and the brain

3: Video games and the brain!

Another technology habit that will RUIN your shot at great sleep, is playing video games before bed.

Most technology based games have time limits, goals with in-game consequences and rewards, and structures intended to keep you playing. They affect your sleep in two ways.

The first way games keep you awake, is by keeping you playing.

Short and simple, game developers want you to stay in their app or playing their game for as LONG as possible.

You are more likely to buy in-game boosters or packages. You're also more likely to see more ads, if they use paid ads. Keeping you in the game is literally a matter of dollars for these app developers, so you can bet they've researched HOW to keep you playing for as long as possible. It's done by making rewards exciting or giving you powers for certain levels of progress.

We've all had that feeling of playing a game and getting more coins, more points, more kills or more resources. It's addicting and we like seeing our 'score' or our numbers go up. The game often rewards certain milestones with encouraging sounds or visuals, to make you WANT to keep playing to get more of that feedback.

It's addictive and keeps you wanting to play. Social media also uses this powerful gamification to keep you scrolling LONG after you should have put your phone down.

The second way games can keep you awake is by increasing the activity in your adrenal system. Your character almost dies in the game and - whoops! Your body gives you a quick spike of *adrenaline*.

Your brain chemistry can't easily differentiate between a real-life threat, and one in the game...

Some games, like solitaire, that have short rounds and no humanizing qualities (no characters, violence or plot), aren't as bad. They can still spike your adrenal system or keep you up late, but it isn't as likely. Overall, the best course of action is to skip all video games for the hour before bedtime.

The worst games for this are immersive free roam games where you're IN the world exploring it, or shooting games. Shooting games tend to raise adrenaline levels and keep you on the edge of your seat. Sure, there are addictive properties of most games, but violent or highly engaging video games are the worst.

You don't have to cut them out entirely, just be aware that they're addictive, they don't really benefit you in any way. They're actually just benefitting the game company, and making them a bit richer.

I won't go into the consumer vs producer mindset in this ebook, but just be aware that you're not really adding anything to your life by playing video games all the time. Try and cut down playing time in the evening and turning off ALL screen two hours before bed.

Using the BEST alarm in the morning

4: Use the best alarm in the morning

People who stick with an old-fashioned alarm clock are one step ahead of the pack. Alarms that don't have a snooze, function and don't produce blue light (or any light with the exception of sunrise alarm clocks if you don't get natural sunlight) are best.

This may mean an LED clock on which you have turned off the sleep timers. Make sure it has a red or orange display. You can also use a manual alarm with bells and a switch. Either of these options is better for your sleep than using your phone as an alarm.

Using your phone as an alarm creates the temptation to check the time whenever you wake up. The same compulsion to answer texts and check on notifications is there, whether it's 3PM or 3AM.

When you wake up in the middle of the night and look at the time (and the majority of people who struggle to sleep well wake up during the night), that feeling comes into play. You are likely to get drawn into your phone and start to wake up, rather than going back to sleep.

We've covered phones already, but specifically, think about getting a sunrise alarm clock. If your room or house doesn't get much natural sunlight, or if you need to wake up BEFORE the sun rises, these are perfect.

It's essentially like a normal alarm clock but it slowly increases the brightness on a 'sun simulator' bulb. It lights your room up slowly over the course of about half an hour, to simulate the effect of the rising sun.

There's not much point using these if your room already gets sunlight, but for dark spaces they're GREAT. They're also very useful for waking up naturally BEFORE the real sun has actually risen.

I've used these for years and in Winter especially, because the sun doesn't rise until much later in the day. They'd also be great for people living in places where the suns patterns are annoying or strange..

Places near the North pole like Scandinavia and Canada, sometimes can have MONTHS of no sunlight or MONTHS of constant sunlight.

Place distractions
out of reach

5: Place distractions out of reach

The objects near your bed are important. If you have too many distractions near your bed, it can be tempting to wake up or check things on your night table.

Things like Kindles, books, phones and laptops should be left AWAY from your bed at night!

Try leaving your phone in a different room once you start your bedtime routine (We'll cover routines later). This will decrease the temptation to check it over and over. It will also lower your exposure to blue light.

Turn off the ringer and alert tones and plug it in to charge in your kitchen or living room. You can still use it as a backup alarm - if you miss your first alarm, when your phone wakes you up you will have to get OUT of bed to turn it off.

If you have a job where you are on call some nights, still place your phone out of reach of your bed. This will still negate the temptation to check your phone, and lower your blue light exposure. You will also be more awake if you have to get up to answer a call, because you'll have to physically stand up to get it.

For many people, just changing your technology habits will improve your sleep. A change in habit like this takes up to seven weeks to take effect, though, so don't give up if it isn't effective immediately.

In fact with all of these tips, bear in mind that change won't happen overnight. You'll probably need to give it some time to work, and habits are not easily formed either. These are all habits and good habits are HARD to form, but easy to live with once they're formed.

Bedrooms are ONLY *for sleep*

6: Bedrooms are ONLY for sleeping

You might have underestimated the importance of having a place that is just made for sleeping. For many, especially those who don't live alone, the bedroom serves a number of purposes.

It is a place for reading, TV, phone calls, video games, getting ready for the day, writing or playing games, and finally sleeping/sex.

The problem is, humans are considered "den" creatures like bears. We are naturally designed to have a space for sleeping that is designated for just that purpose. It satisfies an innate need for security while vulnerable.

Turn your bedroom into a place where sleep is prioritized. If possible, move games, TVs, and other entertainment to the living room or a different part of your home.

If they need to stay in the bedroom, make a point of making a place to sit or lay while using them that isn't the bed. The whole bedroom, or at least the entire bed, should be centered around sleep.

This is one thing that can really make a difference. If you take all the things that don't need to be in your room out, you'll be more relaxed when trying to sleep. In fact, your room should be a perfect place to sleep.. You should have incense, dimmable lights, relaxing ornaments and even plants.

I like to have several plants, soft things like cushions, wall tapestries, and inspirational posters in my room. There's not much else that could distract me.

The bed especially, is only for sleeping or having sex. It's never a place to work or read. Begin to build the link between sleeping and your bed!

Sure, it's comfortable to read on your bed, but what you're doing is telling your subconscious mind that your bed is for sleeping AND reading. So sometimes, you'll be laying there trying to go to sleep and your brain wants to read a book!

Start weakening the mental link between your bed and things like working, reading or watching TV.

This is one that will be hard to change if you've always used your bed for such things. It's a habit, and bad habits are always hard to change.

Start with small steps like taking one thing out of your room at a time. Or if you normally watch TV in your bed, physically REMOVE the TV from your bedroom. It's a lot harder to go back to previous habits that way.

One of the most powerful ways of changing bad habits is just to physically remove temptations. If an alcoholic has no drinks in the house, he's much less likely to drink. To drink would involve physically walking to the shop etc...

So remove TVs from your room, make your bed a place of sleep and sex only. After a few weeks your brain will strengthen those links and you'll naturally feel tired just by laying down in the bed.

7: Cool yourself down!

In nature, it is warmer during the day and cooler at night (usually), just like it is light during the day and dark at night. Both of these natural cycles play into what is known as the circadian rhythm.

This is your body's natural cycle of sleep and wakefulness. You can use this to your advantage by creating this cycle within your own home, and following the suns movements as much as possible.

If you want to augment this effect, you can take a hot bath before bed. This is great for those nights where you really need a full night of sleep, like before an important meeting or event. You can also set up a fan in your room aimed at or near your bed to create air flow if you don't have air conditioning.

Aiming the fan right at your face may incite an increase in nasal drainage however, so try different angles to find the perfect position. The exception to this is to have COLD showers first thing in the morning which give your body a boost of 'wake up' hormones,, but most people find cold showers very uncomfortable at first.

Studies have shown that our bodies decrease in temperature as we enter deeper stages of sleep.

Temperature is always linked to sleep, and in general, you want to be slightly colder as you fall asleep.

Try sleeping without socks on, or with a window slightly open. The slight decrease of temperature will massively help your body fall asleep. More importantly though, a well ventilated room can help you STAY asleep for the whole night.

Most people that are interrupted during their sleep wake up because they were too hot. It's so common, and there aren't really any solutions for it either! Unless you have air conditioning, you're at the mercy of the temperature of the room. There is one thing you can do to make airflow better though..

Your *mattress holds the key*

8: How your mattress holds the key

Your mattress and bed make a difference to your sleep.

Specifically, to keep yourself cool during the night, you should remove all clutter from underneath your bed.

Mattresses need to be able to ventilate, and they do this by allowing air to pass underneath the bed and through the mattress from below.

If however, you've got loads of JUNK and storage boxes under your bed, the mattress can't ventilate and you overheat! Try removing all the clutter from under your bed, or raise the bed slightly so air can move under the bed!

I used to have LOTS of junk under my bed but I read a few articles about how this can stop ventilation, and I tried clearing it out. It made an almost instant difference.

I didn't overheat, and my body temperature stayed at
normal levels for most of the night. This makes the
biggest difference in Summer. In Winter, it's not as
important because you'll likely have the heating on
anyway, because you're too cold.

But in hot countries, or in Summer this can really
make a big difference to your sleep quality. It helps to
have a bed that's raised off the ground.

I know there are pros and cons to raised beds vs
futons and lower lying beds, but I've found raised
beds are easiest to sleep in.

Inclined bed therapy

9: Inclined bed therapy

This is something that most people haven't actually heard of. The idea is that by raising one end of your bed up slightly higher than the other end, you improve blood flow and digestion.

This in turn helps you avoid things like Insomnia and acid reflux in the night. The ancient Egyptians used to do this, and they raised the bed by about 4-6 inches.

Importantly, you need to raise the HEAD section of the bed, not the foot section. Raising your head slightly above your feet helps with all sorts of things like blood pressure, digestion, blood circulation and more.

This is a great tip because you can actually do this for free. I did it with some thick old books that I've read dozens of times. Just stick them under the posts of the bed, and you're away! The best benefits are found when you raise the headboard section of the bed by about 6 inches.

One thing to be aware though, is that you'll probably have a double bed with a supporting post in the middle, under the mattress.

It's critical that you ALSO raise this post up, otherwise the weight of your body could break the bed in the middle! Just check that under the mattress, the middle strut is still supporting the weight. I used an extra couple of books and adjusted the strut to be further down.

I'll be honest, it doesn't really FEEL very different to normal bed angles. The real effects are felt after a few nights. You'll notice that you don't wake up as often in the night, and you'll never have acid reflux if you've eaten too much.

Another benefit is that digestion is 10X easier. You'll find you wake up feeling peaceful and regenerated, and you're ready to eliminate waste from your system soon after, like clockwork. It helps food pass through your digestive tract through the use of gravity!

For people who find going to the toilet difficult or you experience digestive problems, this is very useful. I find that since going plant based (Vegan) I haven't really had any digestive issues, but I used to before. It can help the food to pass through your system using gravity to move it down!

With some of these things, when you actually hear it explained you think 'Oh, of course! Why didn't I think of that?'.

But sometimes we just don't think about what we're doing, and whether it's the BEST way of doing something. Inclined bed therapy is something that I remember thinking 'oh, of course!' when I heard about it.

Keeping things clean

10: Keeping Things Clean

Not many people can deny the pleasure of slipping between the sheets of a clean, freshly made bed.

There's a reason for this enjoyment - scientific studies from American universities have recently shown that cleanliness is one of the factors that affects our sense of safety and well being.

Changing the sheets once a week and making the bed daily will help you to fall asleep more easily.

You should keep more than just your sheets clean, though. Air out comforters, duvets and blankets, and wash them often. Dry clean only items like featherbeds should be aired out and beaten, and receive a professional cleaning about once a year.

Declutter your bedroom as well. Hang clothes in the closet or put them into drawers so they are out of sight.

Have designated places for everything, and try to use closed storage options so your room doesn't appear overly full or messy. This visual cleanliness will improve your ability to fall asleep with a calm mind.

You can also benefit from cleaning and decluttering your home and work area at large. Clean, organized, well-balanced areas reduce stress levels and make anxiety more manageable.

You can apply techniques like feng shui, or place things where they seem most suitable to you.

A good example of this is the saying 'tidy desk tidy mind'. It hints at the benefits of keeping your work space and bedroom tidy. Your mind like things to be visually clean and tidy (unless you're a messy sort of person).

The exception to this is if you're more of a creative type. Creative types of people like artists and musicians can sometimes think clearer in mess and clutter.

Embrace the darkness

11: Embrace the darkness

Your body produces melatonin (the 'hormone of darkness') and decreases the quantities of stress hormones in the body (which keep you awake) based on light and temperature among other things. Although keeping your bedroom cool will help, it only does half of the job.

The second necessity to fall asleep quickly and stay asleep more deeply, is darkness. Screens, television, nightlights, windows - all of these take away from the natural state of darkness in which you can sleep best. Do what you can to reduce light from these sources.

Screens are an easy fix, turn them off an hour before bedtime. If you're one of those people who needs the TV on to fall asleep, use your TVs sleep timer. This will make sure it doesn't wake you up later with a loud advert. Most TV's made in the last two decades or so have a sleep timer feature.

Check the user manual or the manufacturers website to find out how to use yours. You can also use a sleep timer to help you remember to turn off the TV at a certain time of the evening, so you don't get sucked into watching loads of Friends reruns, and stay up too late.

If you absolutely need some light in your room, stick to warm colored lights, or light yellow/orange nightlights. Windows are easily darkened with black-out curtains as well. These cost about the same as regular curtains, but have a special panel inside that keeps light from passing through.

This is one of those things you can easily change. Go through your room and look for all the tiny light sources. Maybe it's a few LED charging light indicators by your desk, or a crack of light that can come in through the bottom of your door. Change these things! Either put masking tape over the LED lights, turn them off, or move them to another room. Invest a few dollars in a strip that seals sound and light from entering your room through the underside of the door.

Blackout curtains are probably a bit extreme for most people, but they do make a difference. Always make sure to turn your light off at night, and leave your phone either face down on silent, or in another room.

Silence is
GOLDEN

12: Silence is golden

In nature, things slow down and get quiet when it gets dark.

Your body does this too. Surprising noises or continuous noise tend to disrupt sleep. They can interfere with the brain's ability to enter all of the stages of the sleep cycle successfully, *even if they don't actually wake you up.*

Try to make your bedroom as quiet as possible. Get rid of loud clocks, turn off music, and calm pets an hour before bedtime, or leave them in another room where you can't hear them.

The exception here is classical music, which is shown to increase dopamine and induce a "beta wave," or relaxed, state, so you might want to have that on in the background.

If you do need noise (some people can't fall asleep in silence), choose a noise machine that offers white noise or natural sounds (we have some suggestions at the end of the book). Rain, trickling, or other water sounds are soothing options.

Waves on a shore are another option, and some people enjoy the sounds of a thunderstorm. If you don't want to invest in a noise machine, there are lots of free apps out there. You can also use the quiet noise of a fan or air purifier to calm your senses.

The main thing to note, is that sound can negatively impact your sleep quality and make you feel worse. Try and make your room as silent as possible.

Leaving stress behind

13: Leaving stress behind

One of the greatest woes of current generations, is the high levels of stress. Fast paced lives have created the highest stress levels in centuries.

Researchers attribute this to the sense of urgency created by many types of electronic communication and the inability to truly get away from work and social pressures, even when home alone.

Because of this, modern sleepers find themselves waking several times a night with racing thoughts, or unable to fall asleep because their brains are still whirring away.

To combat this, it's best to use a variety of stress-reducing approaches. We've got to be able to disconnect from work and our social life, and switch off, ready for the night.

Some people have tried-and-true methods to reduce stress, like baths, reading, or yoga. The thing is, everyone's different, and everyone has different things that helps them unwind and remove stress.

The one thing that's universal however, that affects EVERYONE in a positive way, is *meditation*. By meditating every day, you massively (and provably) reduce or eliminate stress and anxiety. It's so powerful that the changes it makes can even show up in brain scans.

Not only that, but meditating actually reduces your risk of all sorts of diseases and conditions like Cancer and Alzheimers.

It does this by lengthening 'telomeres', which are the protective caps on the end of your chromosomes.

Meditation has amazing benefits, and it's so easy to start doing it, that's it amazing everyone doesn't meditate every morning! If they did, there would be far less people being treated for mental disorders, depression and other things like that.

You can start meditating very easily, just by setting a timer on your phone, and being aware of your breaths. Focus on your breathing and try counting your breaths from one to ten.

When you get to ten, start at 0 again! It's a very simple technique that lets you meditate, even if you've never done it before.

It doesn't have to be any harder than that. Meditation is a simple and effective habit, that you can learn to do today.

What you'll find when you do this, is that it's very easy to get distracted. Most of us aren't used to thinking about 'nothing' and we'll find ourselves thinking about anything and everything when we try and meditate.

That's fine, and normal, but just remember to bring your attention BACK to breathing any time you find yourself getting distracted. It's actually very difficult to make the internal dialogue and 'thinking voice' go away! But you have to do it, for your health!

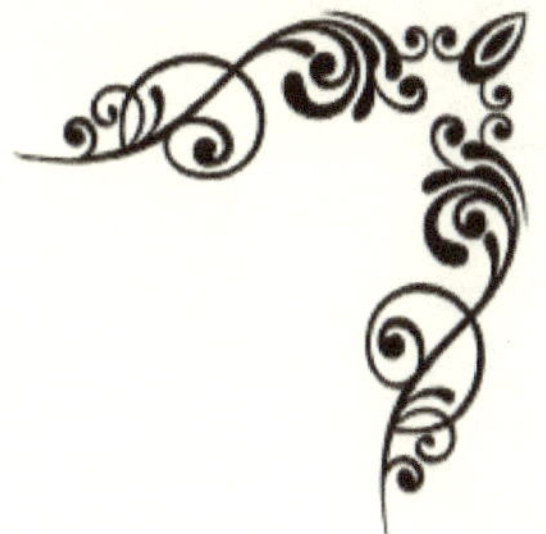

It's all in your mind

14: It's All In Your Mind

Mindfulness is an ancient tradition and habit that still offers a huge host of benefits. One of these is a better night's sleep, thanks to a calmer mind. Mindfulness is literally as simple as it sounds, simply being fully aware; but that doesn't mean it's easy to practice every day.

It takes daily practice. The benefits, however, are HUGE. When you practice mindfulness, you will find yourself falling asleep faster, staying asleep better, and waking feeling more rested.

Try this little mindfulness exercise before bed. Complete it several nights in a row, and you will begin to experience the benefits. You will need a mug of tea or warm milk.

Choose a hot drink without caffeine (which can keep you up) and with little sugar, as the spike in blood sugar caused by the sweetness of soda or honey could interfere with your ability to focus during this exercise.

Start by sitting comfortably in your bed. Many find that sitting against the wall or headboard with their legs crossed is best for this exercise. Pick up your mug and inhale deeply, savoring the smell of the drink. Don't judge whether it smells good or bad, just note that it is there. Review what it smells like. Are there other smells it reminds you of, or is it fully unique?

Next, close your eyes and take a small sip of your drink. Allow it to fill and rest in your mouth. Feel how warm it is, and try to focus fully on the sensation. Consider the flavors:

- How would you describe them?
- Bitter?
- Sweet?
- Citrus or earthy?

Repeat this with several more sips of your drink. You can continue to do so until your drink is gone, if you like. The goal is to fully immerse yourself in the experience of drinking your nighttime beverage. To be mindful and aware.

To be PRESENT.

Next, put the drink down and slide down on the bed, and lay flat on your back on the bed. You can do this under the covers or on top of them. It is important that you lay flat on your back, and not curled on your side or otherwise angled.

You want all of your limbs to lay flat on the bed as well. You should be able to breathe easily, and feel the breath fill your stomach and chest each time. All of your muscles should be able to relax.

Look around your room and consider fully what you can see. Let your eyes linger on shelves, baubles, posters, furniture, pictures, window dressings, and everything else.

Don't sit up to see more, simply look at what is already within view. This likely includes much of your ceiling. Don't pass over it as just a blank surface, consider the details there, too, such as the texture.

Another great place to do this exercise is laying down in a field, looking up at the clouds!

Don't pass judgement on what you see. Simply accept it as what is in your room at the time. Tell yourself it is meant to be there if you are struggling to keep your thoughts in line.

You can also try counting steadily from zero to ten and back, while you look over your room. This will preoccupy the conscious part of your mind enough to let go of other thoughts. If you feel your mind wander, don't beat yourself up about it. Just bring your attention back.

Once you have looked all around your room, reflect on how you feel. You should be able to feel how relaxed you are. Hopefully you are more relaxed than when you began. If not, don't get yourself more stressed over it! Simply accept that it is a tricky night to relax, and move on.

The next sense you are going to use is hearing. Listen to whatever noises you can detect. If you have a fan, this may be the soothing noise of its blades whirring while you lay there.

Keep your eyes closed and keep listening. Can you hear crickets or cicadas outside, or traffic on the street? Listen and give it your full attention.

If a noise like a leaky faucet is keeping you up, find a cadence to its sound. It likely has an exact rhythm. You can imagine a tune to it, or simply give it your full attention. Picture your negative feeling and frustration about it dissipating, allowing the sound to become part of the tapestry of all of the sounds you can hear.

Finally, turn your attention to what you can FEEL.

Consider your weight against the bed, and what parts of your body you can feel touching it. Pay attention limb by limb to how the air and fabric feel against your skin.

Include the feeling of breath entering and exiting your mouth or nose as part of this. Move slowly up your body, thinking about the feeling in your feet, legs, torso, hands, arms, neck and head, until you have scanned your whole body.

By this point, you are likely more relaxed and capable of sleep. Enjoy your slumber, as the resultant shift to beta brain waves and acceptance of noises will help you to sleep deeply, without waking from distractions.

Most people never practice this sort of mindfulness. When's the last time you held your hot drink and took the time to inhale it and focus on how it smells? Or laid there focusing on how the bed feels against your back?

This is the sort of thing you can practice during the day and last thing at night before bed. It works perfectly with normal meditation and relaxation exercises like reading or yoga.

Just breathe

15: Breathe In...Breathe Out

Guided breathing is another excellent technique you can use to get better sleep. There are two different ways you can do this. One is called counted breathing, while the other is cyclical breathing.

Counted Breathing

Start by laying down comfortably in bed. It is best if you are on your back, so that your airway is totally unobstructed.

If this is uncomfortable, try laying on your side with your head on a pillow, so your spine is still as straight as possible. Begin breathing deeply, feeling where in your body your breath travels.

You will probably feel not only your chest rise, but also your upper abdomen and, if you are breathing deeply enough, your belly. Take several breaths like this, simply feeling the air travel through your nose or mouth and into your lungs, then back out again.

Begin counting your breaths, four beats in and four beats out. You can use a traditional method to count, like saying "One mississippi, two mississippi" and so on, or you can simply count at a slow pace.

Do this for twenty breathes, focusing on the feeling of the air travelling in and out, and now on the counting of the breaths as well. This should fully occupy your thoughts.

After twenty breaths, increase the amount of time you are breathing out compared to breathing in by two, you will be breathing in four, out for six.

Do this for another twenty breaths, then progress to four and eight. By breathing longer out than in, you regulate your breathing to match a rhythm similar to when you are falling asleep. This calms the nervous system, sending the signal that, physically, you are ready to sleep.

Cyclical Breathing

This is similar to counted breathing, in that you will measure your breathing. Start out laying on your back, or your side if you need, just like with the previous breathing technique. Start breathing in and out deeply and evenly, feeling the breath in your lungs, filling and leaving your body.

Once you are comfortably breathing regularly, open your mouth a little. Start by breathing in through your mouth, then out through your nose. Do this counting four in and four out. Do this for twenty breaths.

Once you have done so, do the opposite. Breathe in through your nose and out through your mouth. Alternate until you begin to feel calm and sleepy.

Breathing techniques like these are so powerful for improving how you feel, and how you sleep. Most of us don't breathe anywhere NEAR as deeply as we should. Our lungs then start to close up and become weaker! Start practicing deep breathing techniques every day.

I know most people can't practice ALL the techniques and tips in this book. If you can't practice all of them, THIS breathing technique is probably one of the most important ones, certainly in the top 5 to practice.

See the light

16: See The Light (Visualisation methods)

Visualization will also help you to get to sleep. While some visualization techniques common in the Western world involve seeing yourself successful, these do not involve much beyond the image of your physical and psychological self in the present moment.

In this, it is a lot like mindfulness and can be considered another type of meditation.

Peace In, Poison Out

This technique involves picturing the things that do and don't help you sleep, and then exchanging them for another thought. This will help you to mentally prepare for your night. While you do this exercise, try to breathe deeply and calmly.

Start by getting into bed and laying comfortably and untangled, preferably on your back. Close your eyes and think of all the things that keep you awake. Try to picture each one in detail. As you picture each item, turn it into purple smoke.

Continue visualising all of the things that disturb your sleep and your peace until you can't think of any more. Now, imagine this smoke as filling your body, keeping you up. This is the "poison" that you want rid of.

Next, picture all of the air around you filled with golden light. This is the peace that will allow you to sleep. As you picture this light, try letting some of the smoke out of your body to the light and see that it disappears when it touches the light. This is how you will get rid of the things that keep you awake; you will "burn" them away with the light.

Continue breathing deeply. As you breathe out, visualize yourself expelling some of the purple smoke. It disappears when it touches the light. Then, when you breathe in, you are bringing in the light, letting it fill the place you emptied of smoke.

This will be a slow and steady process, not a quick, two minute procedure. When you have finished, you should be picturing your entire body full of golden, calming light.

Safe Space

Think of a location you would very much like to visit,
or one you have been to and enjoy. It might be a
beach, a quiet forest trail, the library- anywhere
peaceful. If you like, you can make one up, but it is
often easier to put yourself into the location when you
have experienced it.

Lay down comfortably and close your eyes. Start by
picturing the place in as much detail as possible. If
you are picturing the beach, you may see white sands
all around you, clear turquoise and blue water, and a
few palm trees.

Be detailed, picturing the frayed leaves of the trees
and lines of shells washed up by the water. Is it high
or low tide? It should be about as clear as if you were
actually there.

Next, place yourself in this scenario. Are you sitting,
standing, or laying down? Explore a little bit, then
find a place in your dream world to lay down and
relax. It should be somewhere you have fully realized.
In your dream world, keep your eyes open, still
experiencing everything.

Once you have found a place, start to imagine the sounds you can hear. Perhaps you can hear the waves rolling into the shore in a soft, repetitive manner.

You might hear the palm leaves rustling in the breeze, and a few birds chirping nearby. Just like with the visual imagery, fully populate the scene.

Now, add smells. Smells are closely related to memory and emotion, and have the power to bring us peace or other feelings. Can you smell the salt of the sea, the brine and sweetness?

Or, can you smell something warm, the sand beneath you? Try to steer away from food smells, as they can be more wakeful and exciting than intended. We all get excited when we smell delicious food!

Finally, add touch. Feel the sand under your back warming your skin, and shifting below you. There's a cool breeze on your face as well.

What else do you feel? The sense of touch is calming, and ties closely to safety in the mind, so it makes it feel like it's ok to rest.

In your dream world, once it is created, allow yourself to enjoy the serenity of the location you have created. Save this as your special place to visit before bed.

When you have rested in it awhile, allow your imagined self to start to close your eyes, and feel yourself get sleepy. As you get sleepy in your vision, you will get sleepy in real life. You should soon drift off to sleep.

Exercising for better sleep

17: Exercising for better sleep!

Believe it or not, physical exercise plays a big part in how well you sleep. If you don't get enough exercise, you will not sleep well.

Increasing your exercise during the day will improve your rest during the night.

(By the way, how are you finding this book so far? If you like it, please consider letting me know what you think!)

There are several different ways to get this exercise. Some of them are better for getting more sleep than others. While there is very rarely anything such as bad exercise, you CAN get too much.

Getting too much exercise, or exercising too close to your bedtime, will make it difficult for you to sleep at night. Instead, make sure that you exercise either early in the morning, or in the early afternoon so that you can sleep peacefully at night.

Really it's about balance. You need to make sure you get enough exercise during the day, but also not TOO much that you're restless at night.

I find the best time to get this exercise is first thing in the morning, or just before lunch.

Of course if you've got a full time job it's harder to decide when you exercise, especially in the middle of the day. If you can decide though, it's best to do it during those times.

But a lot of this is about finding out what works best for you. Some people might get different results exercising at different times, do figure out what works best for you and then do that!

Studies have shown that if you exercise just before a meal, you're more likely to eat the RIGHT amount.

It prevents overeating, which then also avoids things like acid reflux at night and insomnia.

A lot of these things are very interconnected, and if you do ONE thing it can very easily affect other things too. It's also quite difficult to tell which thing or habit

is causing your sleep to improve, so it's probably
better to try these tips one at a time, for a few nights
to really get a feel for what works best.

Yoga for resting

18: Yoga for Resting

Because yoga, meditation, mindfulness, and stress reduction are also closely tied together, most people have some idea that yoga could help them sleep better. However, it is necessary to be sure you are doing the right kind of yoga at the right time of day.

Some Yoga workouts are more strenuous than others. These should be done during the day. If you do them too late at night, you may be kept awake because you have too much energy left over from your work out.

At night, restorative yoga poses are much better to use than other types. Try poses like the forward bend and the lizard pose.

You are choosing poses that increase circulation and stimulate the parasympathetic nervous system, a system largely responsible for low stress and good sleep. These poses also tend to create a calmer state of mind.

If this kind of yoga sounds like a good idea to you, but you think you need to start with something simpler, try stretching every night before bed. Relaxing and releasing all of your muscle groups will ease your body similarly to yoga.

This will help you to get ready for bed in the same way. When you feel you are ready, move onto true yoga poses, or try a simple series of poses.

Just stretching every morning and night will make a difference too, actually! It's well known that most of us don't stretch at all, and it is important.

It's good for your muscles and tendons, and it helps you stay more nimble during the day. It's also important at night, because it triggers a relaxation response in your body.

Try spending a few minutes every evening either doing a light yoga workout, or just stretching and flexing your limbs!

Wear yourself out

19: Wear yourself out!

One of the best ways to get better sleep is to wear yourself out physically and mentally during the day. Those who work in highly physical jobs tend to self-report better sleep.

People like waitresses and construction workers typically state, when asked by researchers, that they sleep well because they are very tired by the time they get home.

You can take advantage of the same phenomenon by getting a good workout most days of the week (without overdoing it). Make sure you still take a rest day here or there so that you don't over exert your body.

You probably think of cardiovascular exercise first whenever you think of wearing yourself out. You're not totally wrong. Cardio is a great way to burn energy, burn off excess calories, and improve your circulation, all of which in turn will improve your sleep.

Cycling is one great option for this. If you bike outside, you get the extra benefits of exposure to nature and fresh air, which also help you sleep better as you read earlier.

Another great cardiovascular exercise to help you sleep better is swimming. Swimming is very easy on the joints, however, it improves long and respiratory health. It also supports health of the cardiovascular and nervous systems. Because most people tend to associate water with calm, peace, and relaxation, you may also feel less stressed after you swim.

Just because cardiovascular exercise is the first thing to come to mind, though, don't discount weightlifting and anaerobic exercise.

These types of workouts often have less of a strain on the joints. They also have excellent long-term effects, like increasing bone density and increasing overall wellness, because increased muscle mass burns more calories throughout the day.

Try basic weightlifting exercises like curls and presses, or squats on the legs, and see what you think. However, just like with rigorous cardiovascular exercise, be sure to do these early in the day. Leave at least three hours before bedtime to relax and unwind after working out.

More than anything else though, focus on cycles. During the day is your time to GIVE and EXERT yourself. Give everything yo've got, mentally and physically and do every task to the full.

Be glad to have the opportunity to do extra work, like walking across the room to get something for someone, or walking to the shops with someone just for those extra steps.

It will all build up and eventually by the time it's bedtime, you'll be VERY ready to sleep. Your body will be crying out for sleep and you'll be able to fall asleep pretty instantly.

Routine is KING

18: Routine is KING

In the race for the best sleep, routine and habits win every time. Good sleep is the result of good habits. You already have a great idea of how the habits of exercise mindfulness and good hygiene will help you sleep better.

However, you also need to have a great bedtime routine. You should try to stick to this routine at least six nights a week if not every night.

Start your bedtime routine roughly an hour before you plan to try to fall asleep. If you want to get eight hours of sleep, and have to be up at 6 AM, then you need to be asleep by 10.

That means you should start your sleep routine by at least 9 o'clock at night. A good sleep routine is typically made up of activities that are calming, like meditation or reading.

Do not eat in the hour before bed, unless you have dietary needs that require you to do so. Putting down the fork should be the beginning of your nighttime routine. As soon as it is roughly an hour before bed, go ahead and start getting cleaned up for bed.

Just like sleeping in clean bedding and clean pajamas will help you sleep better, having a clean body will also help you to sleep well. Wash your face, if not your entire body. Be sure to brush your teeth as well.

After you get cleaned up, and changed into your bedclothes, go ahead to the bedroom. This is the point at which you take the dogs out for one last time, if you need to make sure your pets are taken care of.

Now try and read something. This may be something like the same novel that you read every night, or the same magazine. As you read before, try to avoid reading on screens that use blue light. Reading a paper book, or a book with a blue light filter is best.

You could also apply some of the mindfulness or meditation techniques from this book, or do some mild stretching.

Many men and women also like to include a thorough skin care routine at this time. If you include soothing music and use products that smell nice, your skin care routine can be part of the soothing pre-bedtime routine.

Don't forget, your routine doesn't have to ONLY be during the evening. You should make sure that you are going to bed at the same time every night. Try not to change this routine time by more than an hour on every given night.

You should aim to wake up at the same time every morning as well. This will help your body to know when it should be at certain points of your sleep cycle.

Waking up at the wrong time during your sleep cycle will make you feel groggy and unwell. Some people call this a "sleep hangover".

You should aim to wake up at the same time every morning as well. This will help your body to know when it should be at certain points of your sleep cycle.

A powerful tip for this, is to NEVER go back to sleep if you wake ups bout half an hour before your alarm goes off. Our sleep cycles last 90 minutes, so you'll get woken up in the MIDDLE of the sleep cycle if you snooze for half an hour. Trust me, it's not worth it, and you'll feel 3 times as tired if you do that!

If you naturally wake up a while before your alarm goes off, just go with it. Get up and go about your day, and don't go back to bed to snooze!

One of the most powerful tips for success in life, is to plan out your day the night before. It's easy to do things the next day if you've already planned them out, and you already sort of know what you're doing.

Start writing down a few things you'd like to get done the following day in the evening. Leave it as a note on your desk or something like that, and then when you wake up, do those things!

Using sleep aids

19: Using sleep aids?

If all else fails, you can indeed go to the medicine cabinet. This still does not mean that you need to get into any fancy drugs. There are a wide variety of herbal supplements and teas that you can use to improve your sleep.

Many of these need only be used for a short time to be effective. Their effects will last long after you have stopped taking them, even to an extent of months or years. They can often be used to simply reset your sleep schedule and synchronize your self to your necessary sleep cycle.

For the record, we don't advise using sleep aids most of the time.

This is for those who need an instant boost at the start of their journey. If you're just starting to improve your sleep, a natural sleep aid can help you but we suggest getting OFF them as soon as you're able to.

Kava Kava

20: Kava Kava

This is a great natural sleep aid, but it can be hard to find.

Kava root has been used in the Pacific Islands for centuries to improve sleep. It is a sedative herb. While some people do benefit from taking during the day for anxiety, it is too powerful to be used consistently for that purpose.

However, this strength makes it a great choice for bedtime. It is usually made into a tea.

Drink a mug an hour before bed. It may take a week for kava to start being fully effective. Do not use this for more than six months at a time, though.

Sleep teas

21: Passion Flower and 'Sleep Tea'

One of the most widely studied sleep aids from the natural world is the passion flower. Passionflower, according to many German studies, is proven to improve the quality of sleep, and to help people STAY asleep.

Use passionflower when you find yourself waking up in the middle of the night often, or when you're racing thoughts keep you from falling asleep or staying asleep. This is another herb that you should not use for more than a few months at a time.

Many tea companies offer a herbal tea blend they call a 'sleep tea'. Passion flower is a common ingredient in these teas, so make sure you are not getting too much.

While it is hard to overdose in a short time span, it is possible to drink sleep tea for months on end because you enjoy it, and not realize how long you are using passion flower for.

These sleep teas can also be found without passionflower, and instead include ingredients like Rosehip and chamomile.

Using melatonin

22: Melatonin: Is it really effective?

Melatonin is perhaps the most common sleep aid used in most first world countries. Melatonin is the chemical/hormone made by the brain when the circadian rhythm suggests that it is time to sleep.

Your body naturally makes this hormone, but for some people it's confused or doesn't produce properly. Especially for people who work nightshifts or have a bad sleep schedule, using melatonin can be essential for getting to sleep on time.

Melatonin encourages the parasympathetic nervous system to calm the body and prepare it for the complicated recovery process that happens overnight.

Melatonin is safe to take long-term, provided you don't overdo the dosage. This is one reason it is so commonly used. However, you should still take the lowest possible dose of melatonin to get the effect that you need.

Don't look at the time!

23: Don't look at the time

We've all done it. you're laying there having just woken up at a random time, and you check the time. It's 3AM! Why aren't you asleep?!

Looking at the time just further reminds you that you're not falling asleep, and you've got work in 5 hours. It's just going to panic you and make you stress out even more.

Hide the clock and don't look at it at all! Not even a glance at your phone. Just relax.

The best way of actually doing this, is to remove your phone from near your bed as we've said in previous steps.

It's easier said than done, because most of us are addicted to checking our phones. Try really hard to remove your phone from your room though!

Also, what you can do is get an alarm clock that doesn't show the time on the screen, or one that you can turn the screen off. This means you won't be able to check the time and freak yourself out thinking 'I should be asleep by now!'.

The best ones are actually the sunrise alarm clocks, because most of them come with the feature of being able to turn off the display if you don't want to see it.

Wear your socks
to bed

24: Wear your socks to bed

Science has proved that in order to experience rapid sleep onset (fall asleep fast) your feet and hands need to be warm.

You may have noticed that you naturally try and warm up your chest and hands (and you wiggle your feet) when you're cold and trying to fall asleep.

Wearing socks keeps your feet warm and makes you fall asleep faster, so it's worth a try.

Don't confuse this with the earlier step, which was to make your body COLD. The body needs to be suitably cold in order to enter deep sleep faster. You can make your body cool, while your feet are kept warm by socks though!

This is another one that's quite personal. Some people really feel they can't fall asleep with socks on, while others think it helps them.

Most of these sleep tips apply to everyone, but this one is a very personal thing. Try it out and see how you feel. If you don't think it's helping you, or you think it's keeping you awake, just don't do it any more.

I find that this really also depends on the season. for example in Summer, I can't sleep with anything on, but in Winter it's easier to fall asleep with socks on, otherwise your feet get too cold.

It will depend on the temperature and weather where you live, and what time of year it is. In general, we shouldn't be leaving our socks on, because our feet need to breathe!

But for some people, leaving socks on can make it easier to fall asleep, so try it out.

Dunk your face!

25: Dip your face in freezing water

Submerging your face in cold water triggers an involuntary response called the 'mammalian dive reflex', which will help you control your nerves and it relaxes you. It sort of resets your nervous system.

Do this just before going to bed, and you'll notice that your entire system just feels more relaxed!

This actually ties in with cold water therapy which we'll cover in much more detail later in this book. Just by submerging your face in cold water before bed, you'll notice it's much easier to fall asleep.

In fact, you can do this in the morning as well, to wake yourself up.

It's strange that doing this can both make you fall asleep faster, AND wake you up, sort of like a paradox.

Be careful with this one if you're not used to cold water, because it can be very hard to experience cold water at first. In fact, a lot of people when they first do this have the urge to flinch and even panic and inhale sharply. Make sure you do this slowly, and start with tepid temperatures at first.

Don't just jump in with the coldest water you can get, because you might accidentally swallow some of it! The same goes for cold water therapy and cold showers which we'll cover later.

But don't be put off, the benefits of doing this far outweighs that little risk.

And like anything here, just start slowly. Don't make all these changes at once! And in particular with this one, slowly decrease the temperature little by little.

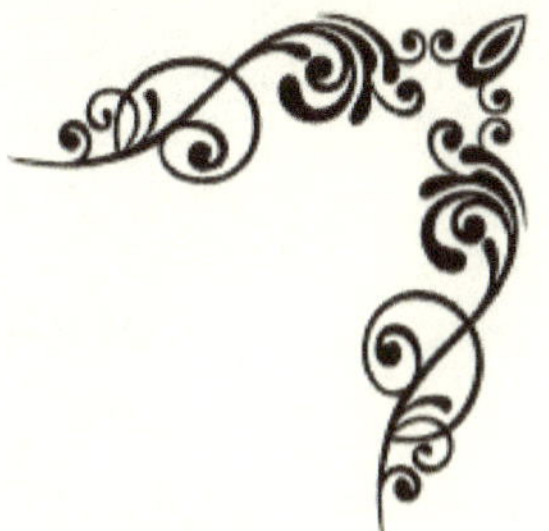

Using binaural beats

26: Try Binaural beats

Binaural beats are a special type of soundwave that
you can listen to, which guides your brain into
various states. They're easy to use, and you can listen
to them through your headphones as you're trying to
go to sleep.

There are lots of different types of binaural beats, and
they all do slightly different things. The most
common ones are for studying, focusing or sleeping.

you can also get binaural beats that make it easier to
lucid dream and do exciting things with your sleep,
but for most of us we just want to fall asleep faster. So
you can actually get packages designed to help you
fall asleep faster, and they're very easy to find online.

The best ones I've used were Ennora, but you can find
others as well. In fact in the bonus section at the end
of this book you can find some links and discounts for
popular binaural beats providers. But in general,
here's how they work:

Your brain can be tricked into hearing a frequency that isn't really there. It works like this:

One frequency is played in ONE ear, while a slightly different frequency is played the other ear. This means there is a very slightly difference in pitch which your brain and ears can't really detect.

So what it does, is slowly change the brainwave state as a result. It's almost magical. Think of it like a tuning fork, slowly making the objects around it vibrate at the same frequency.

Your brainwave state and the frequency of your brainwaves can be CHANGED by listening to certain binaural beats. This is a breakthrough (at least, it was a few years ago) and it's a powerful tool for all sorts of motives.

I like using binaural beats to sleep better, dream, lucid dream, and focus or study. I study things a lot, and I need to be able to focus for long periods of time every day. Binaural beats are great for this, along with nootropics like Mind Lab Pro (links at the end).

Making a dream pillow

27: Make a dreaming pillow

A dream pillow is a special type of pillow that you can create with scents infused in it, which are proven to help you fall asleep faster, and deeper.

You can easily make your own! Sleeping on a dream pillow will make it easier to fall asleep at night.

To make your own, simply order some things like an essential oils kit, lavender oil, and some relaxing and nice smelling herbs. Put them into an old sock or a fabric holder, and let them infuse in a hot place like an airing cupboard or above a heater.

It works best if it's a small thing, like a sock. That way it can fit under your pillow, or you could put it next to a bed. The aromas can infuse better when they're heated slightly.

It's also useful to drip essential oils over it, and around your other pillows.

4-7-8 breathing

28:Use the 4-7-8 method

This is a method of relaxing and breathing that you can do at any time but it's very good for when you're trying to fall asleep and you want more oxygen going to your brain.

There are several ways of doing this, but the principle is always the same: Getting you to slow down your breathing. The 4-7-8 breathing technique works like this:

- Breathe in for 4 seconds slowly, through your mouth
- As you're inhaling, press your tongue against the roof of your mouth
- Then hold your breath for 7 seconds or so
- Exhale slowly for 8 seconds and repeat this
- It might feel difficult at first, if you're not used to doing this! Be patient and if needed, start off with smaller times!

It's a fantastic way of staying focused, and improving your breathing. As I've said, hardly ANY of us breathe as deeply as we should. Our lungs become weak and less powerful. By practicing techniques like this, you can actually improve your lung capacity over time as well.

No heavy foods

29: Don't eat heavy foods just before sleep

Eating foods that are considered 'heavy' or hard to digest can make it much harder to fall asleep on time. Try limiting your LAST meal of the day to something light and easy to digest like carbs or vegetables.

Lots of protein (meat or eggs) will make it harder to sleep because your body will be trying to digest the protein! It also increases chances of heartburn! I'm not going to go too much into diet, but having a vegan plant based diet will really help you sleep better.

It's hard to say which things had which effects, but around the same time I went Vegan I noticed an improvement to my sleep.

This was also the time I change other things like sleep habit etc, but it's still a good thing to try.

Plant based meals are much easier to digest, and our bodies are physical designed to digest plant based foods. They're not designed to digest things like meat!

If you look at the intestines of a human compared to an actual carnivore like a Tiger, there's a big difference. The tigers intestines are short, and the meat quickly passes through the animal before the meat can decompose and rot.

In a human however, the intestines are much longer and food sits in there for much longer. Meat when left in the intestines just rots and purifies, causing all sorts of inflammation and disease.

But that's another topic, you can research that one for yourself. In general, a plant based diet makes it easier to sleep.

Have a massage

30: Get your partner to massage you

If you live with a partner, get them to give you a short massage before bed, focusing on the neck, back and shoulders as these carry the most tension. The shoulders and neck especially can hold lots of unwanted tension and can make it harder to fall asleep.

Small circular motions on the shoulders from a partner can help with this!

It doesn't really matter if they don't think they know HOW to massage someone. You can teach them, and there are lots of videos on YouTube showing you how to massage properly. Just rubbing your neck and shoulders will make a big difference!

Try and use some oil or something to make it more enjoyable, and maybe turn the lights down as well. Music in the background makes it more relaxing, And the temperature of the room should be fairly warm, so you don't get cold or uncomfortable.

Another note about tension, is that you often carry LOTS of tension in your jaw and throat. It's often hard to even notice unless you think about it. Right now, focus your attention on your mouth, jaws and neck.

You'll probably notice that you were holding one part of it stiff or in one position. This especially happens at night when we're laying there thinking about things.

You'll find that instead of moving your limbs, you'll actually tense up your jaw in certain ways, as a reaction to what you're thinking about. It's often impossible to notice unless you focus on it, so watch out for that one!

It's important to be completely relaxed when you fall asleep, meaning no tension in any part of your body.

Wear something comfortable

31: Wear something comfortable

Wear something nice and loose when sleeping. Don't try and go to sleep wearing some pajamas that are too tight and restrict movement, and if you feel more comfortable sleeping naked, do it! Just speak to your partner and check they're cool with that!

The thing about clothes is that if you're wearing something uncomfortable at night, it's just going to wake you up in the night. You'll either get too hot, or you'll turn over and get restricted by your clothing and have to wake up to sort it out.

That's why I think the healthiest and most natural way of sleeping is naked, without wearing anything at all. Of course, this might be weird at first, or even uncomfortable if you're not used to it, but it's worth a try.

At the very least, try and change from full length pyjamas to something like boxer shorts, or pyjama shorts. Trousers are often an annoying thing to sleep in, and you'll find you wake up sometimes just because the trousers got tangled as you turned over.

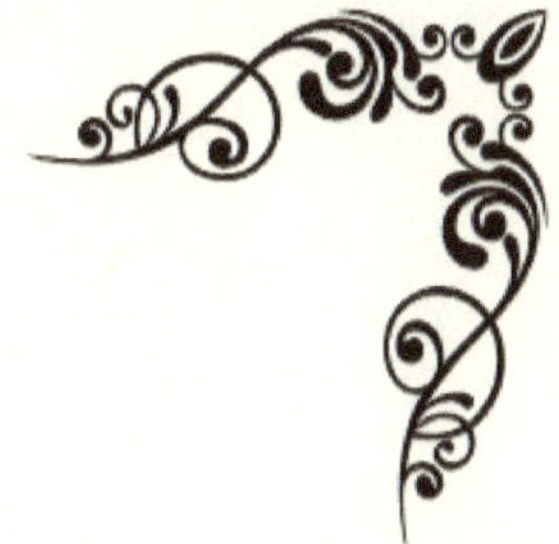

Good posture!

32: Get your posture right

The best posture for sleeping is usually on your side or back with your neck angled slightly upwards so that you're easily able to breathe.

Don't hunch yourself over too much because it's bad for your back! It's important to keep this posture throughout the night, so you can breathe properly the whole time.

It's amazing how many people practically choke themselves in the night because their posture is wrong. Make sure to set yourself up before you go to sleep to sleep comfortably.

Like I said the best position in general is on the side, but some people prefer sleeping on the back and that's fine too, but note that more snoring happens that way.

If your partner snores, it's probably because they sleep on their back during the night without knowing it! Have a go at changing your sleep position and see what a difference it can make.

Get a better mattress

33: Get a GOOD mattress

It can't be stressed enough how important a good mattress really is for the quality of your sleep and dreams.

Memory foam is almost always the best option as it provides great support but also adapts to your body every night. You're asleep for a third of your life, don't cheap out on a mattress!

A lot of people don't think about this enough. You spend hundreds of dollars a month on food, yet a mattress that you sleep in every night for your whole life, you won't spend more than say $500 on!

Having a good mattress makes such a huge difference to how well you sleep!

It's also not that expensive, when you consider how long you'll use it for, and how important is! You can get most high end mattresses on finance, and I think it's well worth it for a good quality mattress, but make sure you really like the feel of it.

Often, the FEEL of a mattress can be misleading. It might be all soft in the show room, but if it overheats during the night, you'll be sending it back for a refund! Make sure you understand how mattresses work, and get one that's not going to overheat during the night.

This is where reading reviews comes in really useful, because you can see what real customers think of things before buying them. Especially because it's so massive, and once it's unfolded, it's very hard to post a mattress back for a refund. So you need to make sure you get a good one, and read reviews before buying.

Especially on Amazon, if the reviews are bad, don't get it. They're almost never wrong, and the reviews are from real people who have really bought it and tried it!

Your sex life

34: Your sex life

Having sex almost always makes you tired instantly after. Use this to your advantage, and have sex with your partner just before going to sleep. For even better results, have sex, then dunk your face in cold water, then meditate, then fall asleep! Works like a charm.

This is a nice way of ending the night with your partner as well. It releases happy hormones and feel good hormones. This makes it much easier to fall asleep!

The only warning with this one, is if the rooms too hot, you can end up making yourself so hot and sweaty that you can't actually fall asleep anyway. Make sure you've got a fan or some sort of air ventilation system before trying this one.

Of course this is an optional one, like most of these tips. Some won't apply to you, some will.

No more naps

35: Stop napping!

Having naps during the day can keep you up at night, if they become too regular. If you HAVE to have a nap in the day time, try and limit them to only in the afternoon, and only for half an hour or so at a time. Never more than 2 hours otherwise you're really stopping yourself from being able to sleep at night.

I've tried various sleep techniques like polyphasic sleep, and napping etc. I've found that you can survive on less sleep at night as long as you do get a good nap in the middle of the day.

The problem I find with this, is that your hormones are all over the place, and your body never really gets in sync with the circadian rhythm.

It's not a great long term strategy, unless you absolutely HAVE to do it for work, or your life schedule. If you have to nap, make sure it's only for a small period of time, like 20-30 minutes.

Also consider the time it takes to actually fall asleep and wake up, so it's never exactly 20 minutes. Bear this in mind if you're trying to nap at work.

In general, napping isn't great, because it makes your hormones go all over the place like I said. The best way of sleeping properly, is just to go to sleep at the same time every night and wake up early at the same time every morning. This means you always get the right amount of sleep, and it's good quality sleep as well.

I have done lots of experimenting with other types of sleep, and I've found this is the best way of doing it. Don't practice things that don't work, and learn from my mistakes!

There are lots of other people who have tried this type of sleep hacking as well, and polyphasic sleep etc. It doesn't really work.

Warm drinks

36: Drink something warm

Drink a cup of tea before bed.This will relax you and make it easier to sleep. Combine this with dunking your face in COLD water, and you've perfectly reset your nervous system and you'll be ready to pass out!

I like to drink something relaxing like decaffeinated green tea. This means it's not going to keep me awake at night, and it's warm enough to relax my body.

The best thing to do actually is to have a cold shower in the evening, and the have a warm drink afterwards.

It really relaxes your system and makes you ready for bed. Be careful the contrast isn't too big though, as it could be shocking or uncomfortable.

Get more SUN

37: Get lots of sunshine

Sunlight during the day increases production of serotonin in the body which is your wake up hormone.

When this peaks and reaches the optimal levels, it starts to actually help make you more tired and you start producing melatonin! If you can, try to wake up with the sunrise, and go to sleep shortly after it sets.

There are actually lots of health benefits to getting enough vitamin D in the day time. This helps you with all sorts of things and it's great for your skin.

Just be careful you don't spend too much time in the sun, because that can be dangerous.

Like with most of these tips, it's all about balance. Spend a bit of time in the sun but not too much. Also make sure that if you're in an area where the sun is hotter, use sun screen to avoid burning and getting ill.

Limit your caffeine

38: Limit your caffeine intake

Coffee is great and everyone likes a cup in the morning. It gets you going, and although it's not 100% healthy for you to have ALL THE TIME it's okay once or twice a day.

The problem is when you drink it 6 times a day and the last cup is with dinner at night! Don't drink coffee or consume caffeine after 3PM!

Caffeine has a 6 hour half life. This means if you drink some coffee at 6PM there's still half the amount caffeine in your system at midnight!

It makes it very hard to fall asleep when you have this much caffeine in your system so late at night. Try limiting yourself to only having coffee during the morning or at the latest, lunchtime.

For many people that's actually a very big change, but I promise you you'll notice the difference. Caffeine makes it almost impossible to fall asleep, and even if you can, you'll be woken up several times during the night as well.

Cut the coffee out, or at least move it to the mornings only. Also, I find the best time to actually have coffee is the morning. That's when you most need it, but even then, don't rely on it too much.

I won't get into too much detail on this one, but caffeine is bad for you! It overloads the dopamine system meaning over time you need more and more of it to get the same effect.

Also by weakening and overloading the dopamine system, you find less enjoyment in the things that are really good for us, like breathing, walking, exercising and eating good food.

It's a very unhealthy thing to consume, but if you have to have some, have one or two cups in the morning.

Definitely try and avoid the really heavy coffees, like the branded ones you get full of sugar and fat in the store. I won't mention any brand names but I think you know what I mean.

Try and have slightly weaker coffee and with no sugar. If you have to have a sweet coffee, don't use sweetener! Its much worse for you than real sugar, so just use real sugar.

Sweeteners contain a chemical called 'aspartame' which is so dangerous and toxic, that if you pour it on the ground in a jungle, ants will walk AROUND it. And they eat anything!

Tense your muscles

39: Tense all your muscles and then relax them

A great way of relaxing and getting ready for sleep is to relax your muscles in series. Start by focusing on your head and then work your way down your body, focusing on each muscle group and area one at a time.

Try and tense them as hard as you possibly can, and then release it to be as relaxed as you can. Doing this for a few rounds at night will massively help you sleep.

It's also a great way of stimulating recovery from exercise at night too.

Be careful you don't tense your muscles too much though, because this can damage them! It's easy to damage your neck in particular by doing this, so make sure to focus on not damaging your neck when you tense it.

Staircase method

40: The staircase technique

Here's a very simple way of relaxing and getting ready to sleep.

- Imagine you're walking down a long staircase
- With each step, imagine yourself getting more relaxed and closer to being asleep
- As you go down each step, tell yourself 'I'm getting more and more relaxed'

You'll find this is a good way of also having a lucid dream. We haven't touched on lucid dreaming too much in this book, but it's an interesting thing to think about. with practice you can learn to control your dreams with something known as lucid dreaming.

It involves practicing various techniques and habits during the day, and then at night you're able to control your dreams and decide what to dream about.

Anyway what you'll find is that by doing the staircase technique, you'll sometimes have a lucid dream accidentally. If you do this, don't worry, it's perfectly safe and natural. You can't get hurt, it's just a way of waking up your mind inside a dream. This means you can do anything you want.

Drink more

41: Drink enough water

Hydration is very important for energy, health and many other things. Make sure you drink enough water during the day and don't cheat!

Don't develop bad habits like forgetting to drink for hours at a time.

Remember, when you feel thirsty, it's too late and you're already dehydrated! Don't wait until you're thirsty, just drink every now and then as a habit!

It's been said that 90% of people are dehydrated at any one time in the world. This is because most of us only drink when we're thirsty.

By the time we're thirsty, it's already too late and damage is being done. Make sure to constantly drink even just little sips if you're not thirty at the time.

It will make you feel better, look better, and sleep better. To help you remember to drink enough, set reminders on your phone to go off every hour reminding you to have a glass of water. Or you could use one of those big water bottles that carry the right amount water to drink for the entire day.

There are all sorts of new bottles and ways of remembering to drink enough, so there's really no excuse now! Make sure to keep it up even on days when you're not really moving around much.

It can be tempting to not drink because you don't feel the need to, but that's a big mistake. It's even MORE important to drink lots when you're moving around lots or outdoors in the sun.

Stop snoring

42: Stop the snoring!

Snoring can seriously stop you or your partner being able to fall asleep fast, so consider investing in a snoring aid that can help you STOP snoring every night! Also, by practicing good breathing techniques you can stop or reduce your snoring!

Snoring is fairly natural and it doesn't really mean anything is wrong with you, but it's often what keeps you and your partner up at night.

In fact, people who snore can often wake themselves up with their own snoring noise. It can be very annoying, and for your partner it can make sleeping very difficult.

I've known couples who have had to sleep in separate rooms because the snoring was such a big issue for them. It can really make sleeping hard, so try and work out a solution.

Often snoring is a result of some bad sleep habits, and sleeping with the wrong position. Try and improve your sleeping position to be on your side with your neck angled slightly up towards the beds headboard. Don't angle it so much that it hurts you though!

There are also lots of natural products you can get like snoring strips and things you inhale before bed, which unblock the airways.

Reset your body clock

43: Reset your body clock

If lots of these aren't working for you, try resetting your body clock. This won't be easy, it really won't. Rest assured though, that if you do this, you'll have a healthy sleep routine, and getting up at the same time (and going to sleep at the same time) will be really easy for you naturally. Here's what you do:

- Pick a wake up time, let's say 6AM
- Get an alarm clock that makes you PROVE you're awake and up
- Every time it goes off, get out of bed as soon as you hear it
- Stay out of bed, no matter HOW tired you are (and you will be tired, for the first two weeks)
- Keep doing it. Don't worry about the time you go to sleep at night, because naturally you'll feel very tired after a day or two and your body will KNOW when to send you to sleep
- It won't be easy but stick with it after a week or two and you'll be an early riser!

There are many ways of waking up really early. I find the BEST and most effective way of doing it, is just to set really big goals for yourself. Think about what you want in life, and then write a big list of goals, but be really specific.

Write things like 'I want to increase my monthly income to $5000 by December' for example. That way you're really specific and you'll start looking for ways of doing that. One side effect is that you'll think 'I should get to work on making that happen!' and you'll wake up earlier.

It helps massively when you have a REASON to get up early. Make a list of things you want to do in the morning to get you closer to your goals.

Even if your goal is just to wake up early so you can go for a run. Lay out your running clothes the night before, and set your alarm for the time!

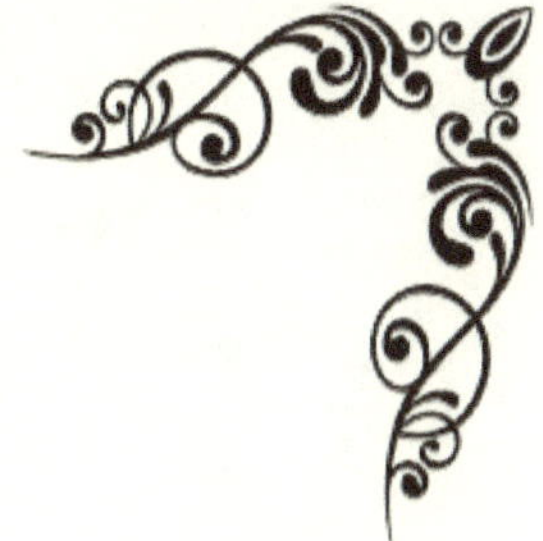

Nostril breathing

44: Breathe only through your left nostril

This is not proven, but some people report that if you breath only through your left nostril by holding the other one closed, you'll feel more relaxed. This is said to only work just before sleep, actually while you're laying in bed trying to sleep. Worth a shot!

I can't really comment on this one, because I've not really tried it enough myself. I think a lot of people find it works, and it's easy enough to try for yourself.

Another thing to consider is that we should really only be breathing through our noses. Our noses are designed to be breathed through, and they have many fibrous hairs along the inside of the nostrils to protect you from inhaling germs.

One of the most common reasons people get colds and other illnesses is that they breathe too much through their mouths. Your mouth is really meant for talking and eating only. You should always try and breathe through your nose.

sleep masks

45: Wear a sleep mask

If there's light coming into your room that you just can't avoid, consider getting a light blocking sleep mask.

This will help you relax and simulate a natural sleep environment where there's no light coming into your eyes.

We spoke about the importance of blocking light from your room as well as sound, right? Well, if you absolutely can't do that, or your partner doesn't want you to do that, a sleep mask is another good option.

The best ones are the sleep masks that wrap around the entire eye, and don't let any light in at the bottom of the mask.

A common problem with masks like this is that you can still very clearly see light through the bottom of the mask with your peripheral vision. Try and find one that wraps all round.

Keep a journal

46: Write in a journal before bed

Writing in some sort of journal before bed can help you get some sort of closure on the day, and help you to leave it behind. If you don't write it down somewhere, it's easy to just keep thinking about it as you're laying there, which of course keeps you awake.

I find it's very beneficial to keep a journal. There are many journals you could try, and I'll link to some of the best ones in the bonus section of this ebook at the end.

To build this into a habit, start writing your day down every night. Just write about how the day went, what went well, and what didn't go well. This helps you reflect and get some sort of closure on the day.

By getting closure on the day, you're more easily able to leave it behind and fall asleep. A lot of people that don't do this find that they're often laying there thinking about the day in their head.

By writing your thoughts down, it's a way of saying 'There are my thoughts, now I'm going to sleep'. It really works as well. In fact one of the most common techniques for dealing with depression, setting goals, remembering dreams or really ANYTHING you want to do, is to make journalling a habit. Writing this stuff down helps your brain process it and make it happen.

Set goals

47: Set goals and follow them

This is actually more of a life pro tip than a sleep tip, but it will massively affect your sleep too. Often, we don't set ourselves goals, and our lives are very much like the same day on repeat.

By setting yourself clear goals and working towards what you WANT in life, things like sleep just fall into place. You'll end up putting more energy out into the world during the day, and feeling more tired at night.

Your body will more easily fall asleep because it knows that you're going to wake up early the next morning and smash it!

If your body works out that you're getting up every morning at 5:30 to smash through your todo list and work on your goals, you'll find it VERY easy to fall asleep at night. I sleep like a rock most nights, and still wake up ver early at about 530AM and work on myself and my goals.

Before I set these goals, every time I tried to wake up early, I just couldn't! I'd always think of a reason to stay in bed that extra hour or so, and in the end I gave up on trying to wake up early entirely. But by having clear goals and a step by step plan for how to achieve them, I'm able to wake up very early with almost no effort.

It's not a chore any more, it's an exciting chance to wake up and take action! It's an adventure, and it really feels like that. But if you're not living the life you want, or you're not trying to change it, you'll find it very hard to motivate yourself to wake up early.

I know this book is about how to fall asleep and get better sleep instead of waking up early, but I think it's ver relevant. By waking up early and working on your goals, you'll also be able to fall asleep much easier at night.

The two things go hand in hand. So take a few hours to really think about your life, who you are, where you're going, and what you WANT. What do you really want?

Maybe it's more money, a better job, a better lifestyle, or even a new partner.

Whatever it is you want, write it down in clear terms and then every single morning, take steps to get to where you want to get! Do that, and your sleep will improve as well, I promise you.

Cold water

48: Cold water therapy

Cold water therapy refers to using cold water to treat various problems. I don't actually like the therapy part of the term, because it implies that you can only use it if there's something already wrong with you.

I like to use cold showers every morning to feel better, and to PREVENT most physical illnesses and problems. By having a cold shower, you get a number of benefits.

The main ones are that you'll feel amazing all day, and you'll have more energy all day long. So that's a pretty big benefit on its own, but there are more.

Our bodies are huge vascular systems. Our bodies contain thousands of miles of vascular cells and fibres, but most of them are laying dormant and not being used.

By immersing yourself in cold water, you force your blood to flow around the entire system. You strengthen your immune system, blood, and muscles.

It's invigorating, and you actually also release certain hormones into your body which are great for health!

But let's not get carried away, it's going to SUCK at first. By having a cold shower, you'll trigger your 'dive reflex' which is the feeling that you need to stop what you're doing and focus intently on the moment.

It stems from when we used to have to swim in cold water to catch our food, or cross bodies of water to get to where we were trying to get to.

Our bodies basically say 'this is cold water, and it's dangerous, let's shut down everything but the essentials and focus on surviving'.

And it lets our blood flow to the important areas. It's a very useful and easy tool for improving your blood flow!

You can have cold showers every day, but I'd suggest just having them in the mornings. A cold shower a day keeps the doctor away!

Get up earlier

49: Get up earlier

We've sort of already covered this one, but by waking up earlier, you do have an impact on your sleep. Here's how it works:

The earlier you wake up, the easier you'll feel naturally tired at night.

If you get it just right, you'll start to feel tired right when the sun's going down in the evening. This is the PERFECT situation, because your body clock is aligned with the natural patterns of the sun.

Your hormones are in perfect balance with when you're waking up and going to sleep.

This is how we were designed to live and function. We should go to sleep when the sun goes down, and wake up when it rises.

We're not nocturnal animals, regardless of how many people think they're 'night owls'. You're not, you've just programme yourself to believe that your sleep DISORDER is a healthy and normal trait.

Humans are not designed to stay up when it's dark. We can't see in the dark, for one! We're designed to sleep when the sun goes down, which is why your body starts producing melatonin when it gets DARK. Melatonin is a sleep hormone that makes you feel tired and ready for bed.

It's so effective, that people actually manufacture and sell it as a sleep aid. But our bodies produce it naturally, if we just got in tune with the sun!

Try it for a month. Go to sleep when the sun sets, and wake up when it rises in the morning. I guarantee you'll feel awesome within a week, and have a lot of unexpected new energy.

Subliminal learning

50: Subliminal learning at night

We've covered a lot of sleep hacking techniques and tricks, but this one's a little different. I've found that if you LISTEN to things at night, some of that information actually seeps into your subconscious mind. I've been able to learn more Italian this way.

I would leave audio recordings of people speaking Italian on in the background and fall asleep.

After a few weeks, I was understanding conversations that were WAY out of what I'd been practicing during the day. I was understanding complex sentence structures that I'd not practiced at all.

And it's because the subconscious mind is like a sponge.

How do you think you learned English?

You just heard it again and again, all day and all night for years. Your mind worked out what words meant, and then with training at school you learned how to form more complex sentences etc...

But the bulk of the work was done just by having people around you speak English. Do the same with whatever language you're trying to learn. Play low volume recordings of the language being naturally spoken all night, and just go to sleep.

Try not to focus on the words at all, otherwise you'll keep yourself awake. Just let the sounds seep into your subconscious mind. To be clear, don't try and listen to the words or work out what they mean!

That's not what this exercise is about. It's about letting your subconscious mind grasp how sentences are formed and how they sound in this language.

Conclusion

If you have bad sleep, don't give up yet. There are so many options to improve the quality of sleep you have every night. While some of these techniques may take a few days or weeks to work, all of them are highly effective. Getting a good nights sleep can make a world of difference in your quality of life. Make sure that you make good sleep a priority.

You don't have to try ALL of the tips in this book. In fact, I don't recommend trying them all. Not all of them will work for you, because sleep tends to be a very subjective thing. What works for you might be annoying for someone else.

For example, background noise! Lots of people SWEAR that background noise is useful for falling asleep, while others can't sleep unless the house is silent.

It changes from person to person, but the one thing that always remains the same is the circadian patterns. Getting in tune with the sun, and when it rises and sets is KEY to getting better sleep.

If you take only ONE thing from this book, it's that. Just follow the sun. Unless of course, you're in a country where the sun's patterns are annoying or unusual, like either of the two poles. for those people, you can use things like sunrise alarm clocks and other devices.

Another thing to consider, is how your overall health is. I've mentioned throughout this book things like meditation, eating a vegan diet, and focusing on your life goals. That's because I truly believe those things are very important. I think they help you do other things, like sleeping better.

In particular, set yourself a life goal. Having clear goals makes it easier to do things like improve your sleep or diet, because you view those things as TOOLS to get to your goals. By having a massive goal, it's very easy to see that waking up a bit earlier every day gives you more time to get there.

It's very easy to eat healthier when you have a huge goal, because you view it as a way of getting more energy and vitality for moving towards the goal. And by goal, I don't just mean what you kinda want. I mean sit down for an afternoon and REALLY think about what makes you tick.

What do you really enjoy doing, and what would you be happy doing if you had unlimited money, OR NO MONEY.

There have been many famous speeches and articles about this topic, but in general, just think about what you want. If you want something that you're not currently getting, you need to DO something you're not currently doing.

And that might include improving your sleep, it might include meditation, or it might be something else. Whatever your aim is, improving your life by focusing on goals will ALSO improve your sleep. Sleep's just a little part of the bigger picture.

That being said, this is a book specifically about improving your sleep, so sorry If we got a little off topic there.

Free bonuses for readers!

It's not quite over yet though, We've come to the end of this book but if you'd like to get a few free bonuses and interesting PDF downloads, head on over to this secret page on my website only for my book readers:

http://www.TranscendYourLimits.com/Bonus

That's it! You have all the tools you need to sleep better, feel better, and have more energy.

The question now is, what are you going to do with
this energy?

*Will it spark a chain reaction that leads to you
becoming the best version of yourself?*

Go and do beautiful things.

You're the first domino..

+++